WƆW

Choosing
a Career in
Pharmacy and in
the Pharmaceutical
Sciences

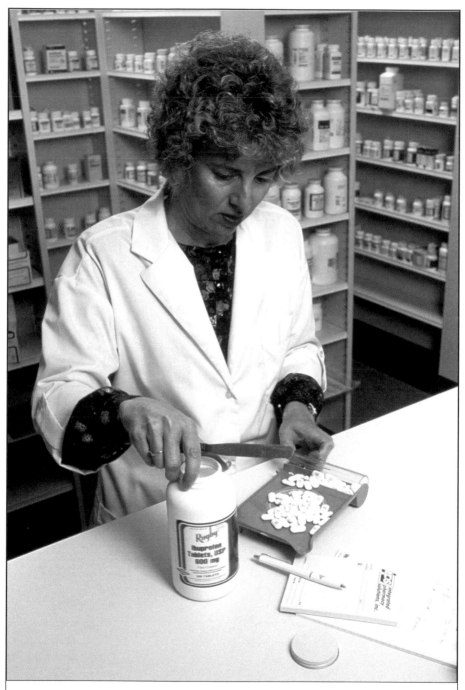

The pharmaceutical industry is growing as more Americans age and need drugs to maintain their health.

Choosing a Career in Pharmacy and in the Pharmaceutical Sciences

Nicole Galiano, Pharm.D.

The Rosen Publishing Group, Inc.
New York

Published in 2002 by The Rosen Publishing Group, Inc.
29 East 21st Street, New York, NY 10010

First Edition

Library of Congress Cataloging-in-Publication Data

Galiano, Nicole.
Choosing a career in pharmacy and in the pharmaceutical sciences / by Nicole Galiano. — 1st ed.
p. cm. — (World of work)
Includes bibliographical references and index.
ISBN 0-8239-3570-1
1. Pharmacy—Vocational guidance.
I. Title. II. Series.
RS122.5 .G35 2001
615'.1'023—dc21

                                        2001004613

Manufactured in the United States of America

Contents

Introduction

Thousands of years ago, way before the invention of modern medicine, people knew that if they were sick, they could use parts of plants or other natural substances to make themselves feel better. In a sense, this was the beginning of pharmacy.

As time went on, people began writing down the recipes for the healing potions that they made by mixing different plant, animal, and mineral parts together. This was the beginning of pharmacy as a profession. There is evidence that pharmacy was practiced as far back as ancient Egypt and ancient China. Just a hundred years ago pharmacists were still compounding (mixing up) most medicines, and they were still using plants and other natural substances in their mixtures.

Today, modern pharmacists mostly dispense medications that are made by pharmaceutical companies, but this doesn't mean that their services are any less valuable than they used to be. There are thousands of drugs on the market today, and modern pharmacists are the only people who have extensive knowledge about all of these drugs. Pharmacists are truly medicine experts.

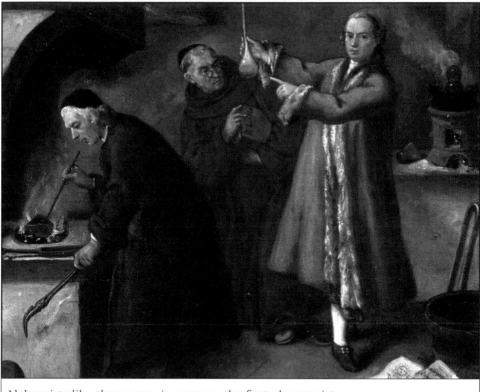

Alchemists like these were in essence the first pharmacists.

If you stop to think about it, modern medicine is an amazing thing. It is incredible to think that less than a hundred years ago people were still dying from simple diseases that can be cured today with just a handful of pills!

If you are interested in the world of science, chemistry, and medicine, perhaps a career in pharmacy is just the job you have been looking for. If, after reading this book, you decide you would like more information about careers in pharmacy, please be sure to check out the resources listed in the back of this book. You will find a list of pharmacy schools as well as a list of Web sites that can provide you with more information about careers in pharmacy.

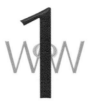

Welcome to the World of Pharmacy

So you think you might be interested in becoming a pharmacist? That's great!

As a pharmacist, you can become a medication expert, making sure that patients get the correct medications, giving out helpful drug information, and helping doctors and other health professionals choose the right drug therapy for their patients.

Or perhaps you're interested in discovering new drugs and medicines that could help people all over the world. Then maybe you should think about becoming a pharmaceutical scientist. Pharmaceutical scientists research, discover, and develop new drugs and medicines that help keep people healthy, stamp out disease, and save lives.

Maybe you want a career in pharmacy in which you can help people, but you don't want to spend years and years in college. In that case, a career as a pharmacy technician might be a good choice for you. Pharmacy technicians help pharmacists provide health care and medication to patients, but they usually only require a few months of training.

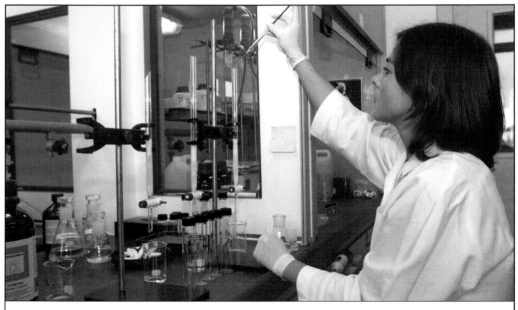
Pharmaceutical research scientists develop new drugs and medicines.

Careers in Pharmacy

There are many different career choices in the world of pharmacy. The purpose of this book is to introduce you to as many of them as possible. You may read this book and decide that you definitely want to learn more about careers in pharmacy. Or, you may read this book and decide that a career in pharmacy is not for you at all! But that's OK—the important thing is to keep researching different careers until you find a job that you think you'll love. As the wise Chinese philosopher Confucius once said, "Pick a job that you love, and you'll never work a day in your life."

There are many different types of jobs available in the world of pharmacy. The three most common jobs in the field are pharmacist, pharmaceutical scientist, and pharmacy technician. Each job has its own unique responsibilities and rewards.

Working as a Pharmacist

Have you ever walked into your local pharmacy and wondered, "What do those people do behind that counter, anyway? Are they just counting pills, or what?" Believe it or not, pharmacists and pharmacy technicians do much more than just count pills.

Pharmacists are medication experts. They are health-care professionals who go to college for six years to learn about drugs and medicines and how they work in the human body. Pharmacists prepare and dispense medications, talk to patients about medicines, give out helpful drug information to patients and health professionals, and help doctors make decisions about drug therapies.

Most people think that pharmacists work only in drugstores, but actually, pharmacists work in many different health-care settings. Did you know that pharmacists also work in hospitals, home health-care companies, and nursing homes? Did you know that pharmacists can travel all over the world working for the army, navy, or air force? And did you know that some pharmacists even work in modern, high-tech laboratories?

There are many different types of pharmacists and dozens of settings in which they work. Let's take a look at the different types of pharmacists and see what they do on a day-to-day basis.

Community Pharmacists

About 60 percent of all pharmacists work in community pharmacies. Community pharmacies include small, independently owned pharmacies, such as local mom-and-pop drugstores, as well as pharmacies in grocery stores, discount stores, and large, national chain pharmacies such as Walgreens, Wal Mart, Eckerd, and Osco.

Community pharmacists have a number of duties for which they are responsible on a day-to-day basis. They fill prescriptions, talk to patients about medications, and answer drug-related questions asked by doctors, nurses, and patients. Community pharmacists also give recommendations to customers about over-the-counter medicines. Over-the-counter medicines are medicines that you can buy in a pharmacy without a prescription.

Community pharmacists also keep medical information about their customers in computers. They use this information to screen (check for) possible drug allergies that a patient may have. They also use the information to see if a patient is taking any other medicines that may interact with the medicine that they are giving to the patient.

Although most medicines manufactured by drug companies today come already put together as tablets, capsules, or liquids, sometimes pharmacists must still compound, or mix up, special medicines. There are even some pharmacies that specialize in compounding.

A Day in the Life of a Community Pharmacist

Some real-life examples may help illustrate what community pharmacists really do on a daily basis. Let's say you're sick. You've been coughing for days, and you finally decide to go to your doctor. Your doctor examines you and decides that you have bronchitis (an infection of the lungs). The doctor then gives you a prescription to take to the pharmacy.

11

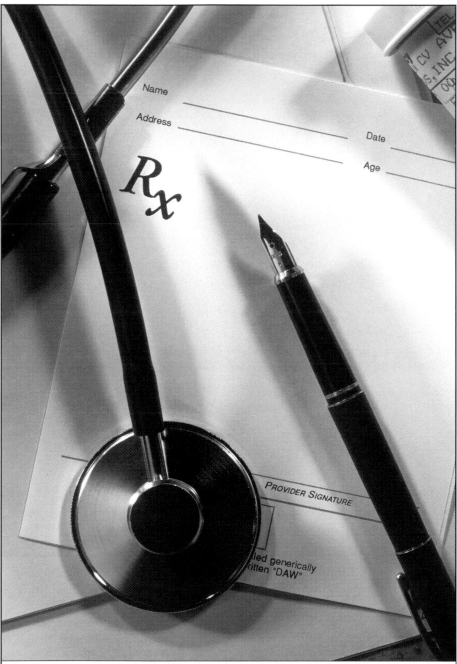

A doctor's prescription contains instructions written in a special code that only the doctor and the pharmacist can read. These instructions tell the pharmacist which medication to dispense and what amount to give.

A prescription is just a piece of paper that has instructions on it for a pharmacist to follow. These instructions tell the pharmacist which medication to dispense. The instructions are written in a special code that only health-care professionals can read. When you get to the pharmacy, you give the prescription to the pharmacist, and then you wait for her to fill it.

You may think that it is taking the pharmacist a very long time just to count out some pills and put them in a bottle, but she is actually doing much more than just counting pills. If you've already been to this pharmacy, the pharmacist has to find your medical information in the computer. She checks your age, your medical history, and whether you have any allergies to any medications.

Let's say you have an allergy to penicillin (when you take penicillin, it causes you to develop a rash), but you forgot to tell your doctor about your allergy. Because the pharmacist is a drug expert, she knows that the prescription your doctor gave you for amoxicillin is related to penicillin. She also knows that amoxicillin will cause you to have an allergic reaction. So she calls the doctor, and together they decide to give you another medicine. The pharmacist puts this new information into the computer. She then tells you how to take your medicine. She also prints out a label with directions about how to take your medicine that you can look at later on if you forget her instructions.

Let's say that you now have questions about your medicine: You want to know what it is and how it works. The pharmacist will then explain to you that your medicine is an antibiotic that will kill the bacteria in your lungs that is causing your bronchitis. The pharmacist might even explain to you that bacteria are tiny little organisms that are too small to see with the human eye, but that cause people to get really sick.

Let's give another example of what a community pharmacist does. This time, it's not you, but your grandmother who gets sick with a bad cold. She wants you to go to the drugstore to pick up some cold medicine for her, but your grandmother also has diabetes, which is a pretty serious disease. To make the situation even more complicated, your grandmother is also taking a lot of different kinds of medications.

You go to the pharmacy to pick up some cold medicine for your grandmother, but on the back of all the boxes of cold medicines there is a warning for a person not to take the medicine if that person has diabetes or is taking certain other medications. Confused, you ask the pharmacist for help. The pharmacist helps you pick out a medicine that will not cause your grandmother's diabetes to get worse, and that will not interact with any of the medicines she is already taking.

Hospital Pharmacists

About 25 percent of all pharmacists work in hospitals. Pharmacists who work in hospitals do things quite a bit differently than pharmacists who work in community pharmacies. These differences in work style mean that hospital pharmacists' jobs are different than community pharmacists' jobs.

For example, instead of reading a doctor's orders from a prescription, hospital pharmacists read orders that are taken directly from a patient's chart. They still enter the orders into a computer, but instead of dispensing medicine directly to the patients, hospital pharmacists dispense medicine to nurses, or into nursing carts. Some larger hospitals even use specialized pharmacy vending machines that dispense medicine to nurses.

Because hospital patients are often very sick, hospital pharmacists spend a lot of time making up IV solutions for patients. "IV" stands for "intravenous," and IV solutions are liquid medicines that are injected directly into a patient's bloodstream. Intravenous solutions must be made in the pharmacy in a very special way in order to keep them from becoming contaminated or dirty.

Working in a hospital can be very challenging and exciting for pharmacists. In some hospitals, pharmacists get to go on rounds with doctors to see individual patients and have the opportunity to answer pharmacy questions asked by doctors and medical students. In some hospitals, pharmacists are part of the medical team that responds to "code blue" situations. A code blue situation is when someone is going into cardiac arrest, and a team of doctors and nurses must work on him or her to get the heart started again—just like you see on television!

In addition to dispensing medicine, hospital pharmacists spend a lot of their time giving out drug information to doctors and nurses. They also monitor the type and amount of medication being given to patients and recommend changes in drug

15

therapy when needed. By doing this, they can make sure that patients are not being given too much or too little medication.

Hospital pharmacists who want to become more involved in hospital administration may eventually advance to administrative positions, such as pharmacy manager and director of pharmacy. These positions offer more responsibility and better pay than staff pharmacist positions.

Clinical Pharmacists

Clinical pharmacists work in hospitals, clinical research facilities, drug companies, health-care clinics, health maintenance organizations (HMOs), and for the federal government. Clinical pharmacists focus more on ensuring that patients are getting the right medication therapy (the right drug, at the right dose, for the right reason) than actually dispensing medications. Clinical pharmacists also monitor lab values and work to reduce drug costs.

A big part of a clinical pharmacist's job is to make recommendations to doctors about patients' drug therapies. For example, let's say that a doctor writes an order for a drug to be given twice a day but the pharmacist thinks it should probably only be given once a day for a particular patient. The clinical pharmacist will then write his or her recommendation on the patient chart, or will call the doctor to discuss the recommendation. A clinical pharmacist might also identify that a certain patient is on the wrong type of antibiotic for a particular infection, and suggest to the doctor a more suitable choice.

Clinical pharmacists also work to identify potential medication problems before they occur. Many clinical pharmacists go on rounds with doctors and medical students, so they are available to answer questions and recommend drug therapies. Clinical pharmacists also spend a good deal of time in meetings with other health-care professionals and hospital administrators.

Some clinical pharmacists specialize in one particular area of pharmacy or work in one area of a hospital, such as cardiology (heart) or oncology (cancer). Some clinical pharmacists even run their own clinics, such as cholesterol clinics, asthma clinics, and smoking cessation clinics. Many clinical pharmacists also publish scientific articles in pharmacy journals, which are magazines that are read by other pharmacists.

Home Heath-Care and Home Infusion Pharmacists

Sometimes a patient is sick enough to need IV medications, but not sick enough to be in the hospital. That's where home health and home infusion companies come in. They provide IV medications and nursing care to patients at home.

Pharmacists who work for home health and home infusion pharmacies prepare IV solutions for patients. Once the solutions are prepared, home health nurses take the IVs to patients' homes and administer the solutions. Home health and home infusion pharmacists also help doctors monitor patients' drug therapies, and help patients and nurses select the proper medical devices and equipment.

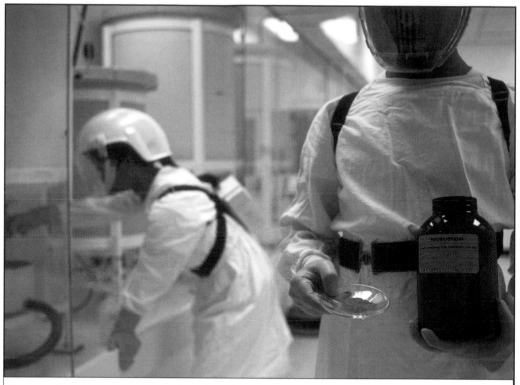

Pharmacists wear protective suits when they work in a "clean room" to ensure that they are not exposed to any dangerous substances.

Nuclear Pharmacists

Did you know that radioactive materials are sometimes injected into patients' veins in order to diagnose certain diseases? Nuclear pharmacists are responsible for preparing these radioactive materials. Some of the more common radioactive materials that pharmacists work with are radioactive iodine and radioactive thallium.

Although doctors use very small quantities of radioactive materials, these substances can be very dangerous. They must be carefully prepared in a special room by a nuclear pharmacist. Nuclear pharmacists often work together with nuclear medicine departments in large hospitals.

Clinical Research Pharmacists

When drug companies develop new drugs, they must first test the drugs on humans to ensure that they are safe and effective. Clinical research pharmacists help to set up these drug studies, and they help administer the drugs to test patients. Clinical research pharmacists usually work for a pharmaceutical company or for an independent clinical research lab.

Drug Information Pharmacists

There are some pharmacists who work full-time providing drug information to doctors, nurses, and other health professionals. They are called drug information pharmacists, and their duties consist of answering questions, evaluating medical literature, and analyzing results from drug studies. Drug information pharmacists usually work in large university hospitals or in pharmaceutical companies.

Because drug information pharmacists work with information technology, they must be very familiar with computers and computer software. Some drug information pharmacists go through an additional year of training, called a residency, to learn how to do their job better.

Poison Control Center Pharmacists

"Help! My baby just drank a bottle of window cleaner! What should I do!?" Believe it or not, this is a common type of question for a pharmacist who works in a poison control center. Poison control pharmacists usually work in poison control centers and answer poison control hotline phone calls.

Pharmacists who work in poison control centers often help frantic parents take care of children who have mistakenly eaten or drank something toxic. They also answer questions for doctors and nurses in hospital emergency rooms who treat patients who have been poisoned or who have mistakenly ingested something toxic. These pharmacists often use special computer software that provides an enormous amount of information about different poisons, chemicals, and dangerous household substances.

Forensic Pharmacists

"Forensic" means having to do with the legal or criminal justice system. Forensic pharmacists are involved in a variety of different legal activities, such as testifying in court for medical cases, helping with the drug testing of athletes, and consulting for lawyers or police. Most forensic pharmacists are part-time consultants who work full-time at other pharmacy jobs. A few forensic pharmacists do work full-time for government agencies, such as the Food and Drug Administration (FDA) or the Drug Enforcement Administration (DEA). Some forensic pharmacists also work for state boards of pharmacy or as forensic toxicologists.

Long-Term Care Pharmacists and Consultant Pharmacists

Nursing homes, retirement homes, and hospices are often called long-term care facilities, because the people who live there often stay for long periods of time. Pharmacists who provide pharmacy care for these people are called long-term care pharmacists.

Many of the residents who live at these facilities are older and sicker than the general population, so they are often taking a lot of medications. In fact, it is not uncommon for one person in a nursing home to be taking up to ten, fifteen, or even more than twenty kinds of medications. Consultant pharmacists help monitor these people's medication therapy. They watch out for side effects and monitor patients for potential drug interactions. They also recommend drug therapy changes to doctors.

Pharmacists Who Teach at Universities

Both pharmacists and pharmaceutical scientists work in many different areas of schools and universities. They work as researchers, professors, associate professors, and assistant professors. Different areas of teaching might include pharmacy practice, pharmaceutics, pharmacology, toxicology, medicinal chemistry, and clinical pharmacy. Pharmacy professors who teach in universities are usually required to have an advanced degree such as a masters in science or a Ph.D. Professors of pharmacy generally start out as associate professors, then work their way up to full professors.

Pharmacists who have a regular pharmacy job, but who also help teach pharmacy students, may be appointed as assistant professors of pharmacy to a university. For example, a clinical pharmacist working in a hospital may be appointed as an assistant professor at a local university, because in addition to doing his or her regular duties at the hospital, he or she is also responsible for teaching pharmacy students during their clinical rotations.

Pharmacists Who Work for the Federal Government

The U.S. federal government employs hundreds of pharmacists. They work in the armed forces (the army, navy, or air force), the Veterans Health System, the Indian Health System, and other federal agencies. Pharmacists in the armed forces have the opportunity to travel all over the world. Military pharmacists serve their country by helping to take care of soldiers and their families in peacetime and wartime. They work in military hospitals, on military bases, and even on hospital ships.

Hundreds of pharmacists work in Veterans administration hospitals, also called VA hospitals. Because military veterans keep health-care benefits for the rest of their lives, there are VA hospitals all over the country. Many of these hospitals are very large, so there are many opportunities for pharmacists to do much more than just dispense medicine. They often work very closely with the patients and the rest of the medical staff. The federal government also employs pharmacists in the Indian Health System (IHS). IHS pharmacists work on Native American reservations. Because these reservations are on federal land, the government often builds health-care clinics on the reservations, and provides the Native American population with free health care.

Pharmacists also work in other governmental agencies in clinical research positions, in administrative positions, and as consultants. These agencies include the Food and Drug Administration (FDA), the National Institutes of Health (NIH), and the Drug Enforcement Administration (DEA).

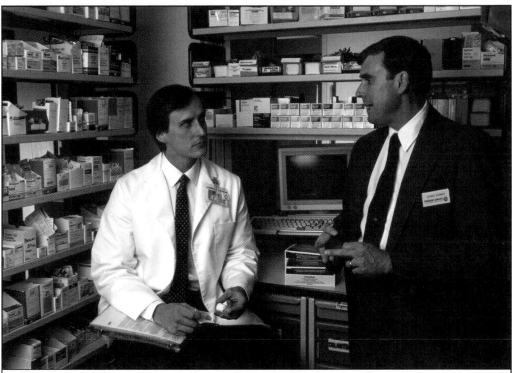

Salespeople from pharmaceutical manufacturers often try to influence pharmacists and doctors to recommend certain drugs to their patients.

Pharmacists Who Work for Pharmaceutical Companies

Although you do not have to be a pharmacist to work for a pharmaceutical company, many pharmacists do. Some earn Ph.Ds and become pharmaceutical scientists. Other pharmacists go on to work in one of the many departments in large pharmaceutical companies. These include sales, marketing, drug information and education, research and development, and public relations.

Other Jobs for Pharmacists

In addition to the jobs described above, there are many, many more positions out there for pharmacists. Some of the other places you'll find pharmacists working in are:

- Pharmacy associations

- Temporary staffing agencies

- State boards of pharmacy

- Health insurance companies and health maintenance organizations (HMOs)

- Medical marketing companies

- Medical education companies

- Drug companies

Working as a Pharmaceutical Scientist

According to the American Association of Pharmaceutical Scientists (AAPS), pharmaceutical scientists develop medicines that enhance life. They are also instrumental in the development of innovative drugs that save thousands of lives and improve the quality of life for many others.

What exactly are the pharmaceutical sciences? According to AAPS, the field of pharmaceutical sciences combines a broad range of scientific disciplines. They are broadly classified into the following categories:

- Analysis and pharmaceutical quality

- Biotechnology

- Clinical sciences

- Economic, marketing, and management

- Medicinal and natural products chemistry

- Pharmaceutics and drug delivery

- Pharmaceutical technologies

- Pharmacokinetics, pharmacodynamics, and drug metabolism

- Regulatory affairs

Pharmaceutical scientists work in three main settings: in the pharmaceutical industry, in universities, and for the federal government. In the pharmaceutical industry, scientists work to develop new drugs, medicines, and pharmaceutical technologies. They work as teachers and researchers in universities and colleges of pharmacy. In the federal government they usually work as clinical researchers (such as at the National Institutes of Health), or as regulatory scientists (such as in the Food and Drug Administration). Because there are so many different jobs, their working conditions and work settings depend greatly on their scientific field and career setting.

Working as a Pharmacy Technician

Pharmacy technicians are vitally important members of the health-care world. They work in many different types of pharmacies, such as community drugstores, hospitals, long-term care pharmacies, home health pharmacies, and nuclear pharmacies. Pharmacy technicians must work under the direct supervision of a registered pharmacist, but in many states pharmacy technicians can do any of the dispensing and compounding activities that a pharmacist can do—as long as a pharmacist checks their work.

In community pharmacies, technicians perform a great deal of the dispensing work, such as picking the right medication off the shelf and counting the pills, so the pharmacist is free to do other things. Often, a technician will fill the prescription and the pharmacist will just check it over to make sure he or she did it right. Community pharmacy technicians also help to enter prescription information into the computer, file insurance claims, run the cash register, maintain pharmacy records, order medications to keep the pharmacy well stocked, and help customers find what they need in the pharmacy.

In hospitals and home health pharmacies, pharmacy technicians help distribute medications to the hospital floors, fill nursing carts, restock nursing supplies, repackage unit-dose medications, compound medications, and prepare sterile IV solutions.

The Job Market, Working Conditions, and Salaries

Now that you have an idea of what pharmacists, pharmaceutical scientists, and pharmacy technicians do, let's take a look at the job market and salaries for each career.

The Job Market for Pharmacists

According to the *Occupational Outlook Handbook*, there were about 185,000 pharmacists working in the United States in 1998. However, there is an incredible shortage of pharmacists right now, so there are many more jobs available than there are pharmacists to fill them. According to a report by the U.S. Department of Health and Human Services, there were about 7,000 unfilled pharmacy jobs in February of 2000.

It is very common for pharmacists to change jobs many times over the course of their careers. Pharmacists will often move from one type of pharmacy setting to another if they get tired of working in a particular place after a while. Also, since pharmacists don't often get salary raises,

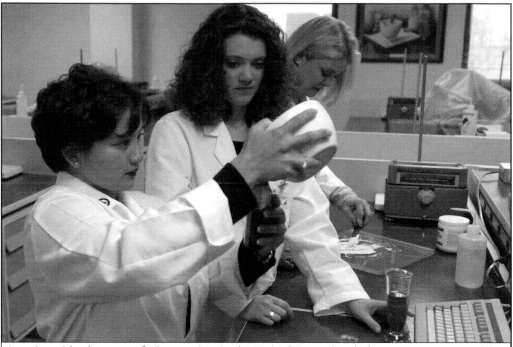

A nationwide shortage of pharmacists in the United States has led to greater opportunities for women and minorities in the field.

moving from one job to another is a common way for pharmacists to increase their salaries. It is also common for pharmacists to work more than one job. For example, they may work full-time in a hospital pharmacy, and then work a few extra days a month in a community pharmacy for extra money.

Hours and Working Conditions for Pharmacists

Work hours for pharmacists vary widely. About 15 percent of all pharmacists work part time, while most pharmacists work full-time. Pharmacists who are pharmacy managers or pharmacy owners often work much more than forty hours a week; in fact, they sometimes even work over sixty hours a week!

Pharmacists who work in community pharmacies tend to work longer shifts than other pharmacists—sometimes ten to twelve hours at a time, and often with few or no breaks. According to a survey conducted by *Pharmacy Week*, 20 percent of all pharmacists report not getting to take any breaks at all during their work day. For these pharmacists, "lunch" can mean grabbing a few bites of a sandwich or chips here or there when it slows down a little bit between customers. In addition, the majority of pharmacists have to work nights, weekends, and holidays since most hospital pharmacies are open twenty-four hours a day, and more and more community pharmacies are open on nights and weekends.

The physical working conditions for most pharmacists are generally clean and safe, and there are not many on-the-job injuries reported. However, pharmacists who work with potentially dangerous materials, such as cancer chemotherapy drugs or radioactive materials in a nuclear pharmacy, must work in a protected "glass hood," and they must wear gloves and other protective clothing.

Salaries for Pharmacists

According to a pharmacy salary survey conducted by *Pharmacy Week* and PharmacyOneSource.com, the average full-time pharmacist's salary in the year 2000 was $74,297. Salaries ranged from $60,000 to $80,000, and were dependent on several factors, including region of the country, practice setting, position, gender, education, and experience. Interestingly, pharmacists who live in the western and southern parts of the United States make more than those who live in the Northeast and Midwest.

Pharmacists who work for pharmaceutical companies made the highest salaries in the year 2000—an average of $80,000. Home health and nuclear pharmacists have the next highest salaries, with an average of $77,000. The average salary for community pharmacists was $74,880, and the average salary for hospital pharmacists was $72,280.

Despite the fact that more women are graduating today from pharmacy school than men, male pharmacists are still getting paid slightly more than women. According to the salary survey, the median male pharmacist's salary is $72,000, but the median woman's salary is only $70,637.

Pharmacists' salaries tend to increase depending on their experience and with added managerial duties. For example, directors of pharmacy and pharmacy managers make more than staff pharmacists, and pharmacists who have gone on to earn a master's degree tend to make higher salaries than pharmacists who have just a B.S. or Pharm.D. degree.

Because of the high demand for pharmacists right now, many pharmacies and hospitals are offering pharmacists sign-on bonuses to lure pharmacists to come work for them. These sign-on bonuses can be anywhere from $2,000 to $10,000. A full 30 percent of pharmacists who have taken new jobs in the past year reported receiving sign-on bonuses!

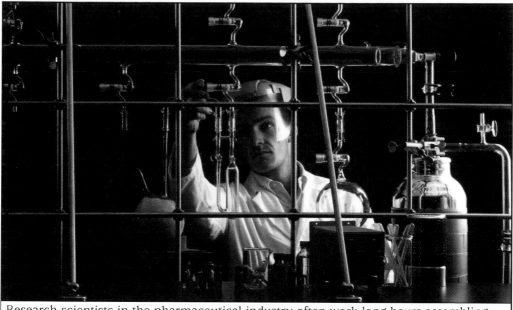

Research scientists in the pharmaceutical industry often work long hours assembling experiments and conducting tests.

Community pharmacists who work for large chains are eligible for extra yearly bonuses, based on the profitability of their store. This can substantially add to their yearly income. Community pharmacists may also be promoted by the companies they work for. Promotions to such jobs as pharmacist in charge, pharmacy manager, and regional manager offer community pharmacists a chance to earn even more money.

Benefits for Pharmacists

Benefits for pharmacists are usually very good. They get paid health insurance, paid vacation time, profit sharing, bonuses, and 401(k) retirement accounts. In addition, pharmacists who work for the federal and state governments often get a minimum of a month's worth of paid vacation each year!

Job Market for Pharmaceutical Scientists

According to the AAPS (American Association of Pharmaceutical Scientists), there are three main areas where pharmaceutical scientists can find jobs: in the federal government; in universities; and in the pharmaceutical industry.

The demand for pharmaceutical scientists is strong right now, although fluctuations in industry hiring trends do occur from year to year, due to industry mergers and acquisitions. For example, according to a salary survey conducted by AAPS in 1999, industry hiring by drug companies declined 13 percent in 1999 from 1998. The planned hiring rate was 9 percent higher in 2000, but no official statistics were available yet at the time of this book printing. Many respondents (28 percent) at the time of the survey indicated that they were considering changing jobs, but this figure was down 4 percent from 1998. This was mostly due to a large number of mergers and acquisitions of large drug companies in the past few years, which would affect their employment security in the near future.

Hours and Working Conditions for Pharmaceutical Scientists

Scientists that work in the pharmaceutical industry usually work for pharmaceutical or biotechnology companies. The exact type of work that they do varies, as do their working conditions, depending on what kind of science they are involved in. For

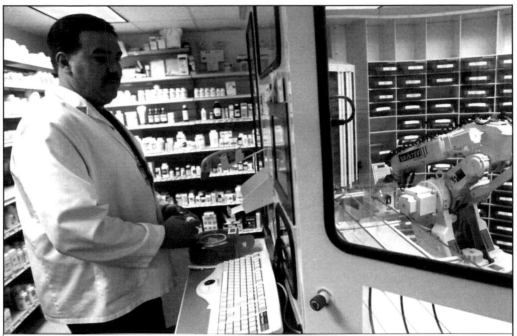
This pharmacy technician is operating a robot that puts various drugs in the correct bins at the pharmacy.

example, a medicinal chemist might be working with lots of technical equipment and machines that measure what different types of drugs are made of, whereas a pharmacologist might be working with animals to test drugs.

Pharmaceutical scientists who work at colleges and universities usually work as researchers and/or as teachers. Most of them, especially those who are working on their Ph.D. degrees or in postdoctoral training, usually work very long hours in their laboratories.

Pharmaceutical scientists who are employed as regulatory scientists by the federal government usually work for large federal agencies, such as the FDA. Their jobs are typically more administrative and are often much different than the jobs of industry or academic scientists.

Salaries for Pharmaceutical Scientists

According to an AAPS 1999 salary survey, salaries for pharmaceutical scientists vary widely depending on the work setting of the scientist. The average salary is around $90,000 a year. The average salaries for industry scientists were $93,000, $85,200 for academia (colleges and universities), and $86,000 for government employees. The average starting salary for a beginning scientist was $60,900.

Individuals with degrees in toxicology were paid the highest, at $103,800, followed by degrees in physical chemistry ($102,000), pharmacology ($102,000), and pharmacokinetics ($101,700). Salaries for individuals with degrees in chemistry ($74,800), biochemistry ($77,700), and inorganic chemistry ($87,000) were the lowest.

Job Market for Pharmacy Technicians

Pharmacy technicians work just about anywhere that pharmacists work, such as community pharmacies, hospital pharmacies, long-term care (nursing home) pharmacies, mail order pharmacies, and nuclear pharmacies. However, the majority of pharmacy technicians work in hospital, community, and home health pharmacies. Pharmacy technicians also work in other settings, such as health insurance companies, drug wholesale companies, and drug manufacturing companies.

Well-trained pharmacy technicians are in high demand today, and the job outlook for the future looks very promising. Because pharmacists have been shifting their focus from dispensing duties to clinical duties, pharmacy technicians perform tasks today that used to be done primarily by pharmacists in the past. Also, as the population in America is growing older, the number of prescriptions filled in pharmacies goes up every year. Therefore, more and more technicians will be needed to help fill all those prescriptions.

Hours and Working Conditions for Pharmacy Technicians

The working conditions for technicians are about the same as for pharmacists. They are often expected to work nights, weekends, and holidays. Technicians usually get more breaks during the day than do pharmacists, however, and they aren't typically expected to work the unusually long shifts in community pharmacies that pharmacists do. In addition, pharmacy technicians don't usually have to work "on-call" hours.

For technicians, the physical working conditions are clean and safe, and there aren't a lot of on-the-job injuries. Pharmacy techs who work with potentially dangerous materials, such as cancer chemotherapy drugs or radioactive materials in a nuclear pharmacy, must also work in a protected glass hood, and wear gloves and protective clothing.

Salaries for Pharmacy Technicians

Pharmacy technicians don't make the high salaries that pharmacists make, but their jobs don't require as much education as pharmacists' do. According to the salary survey conducted by *Pharmacy Week* in the fall of 2000, the median pay for technicians in that year was $10.94 per hour, which equals about $22,700 a year. Well-trained technicians with a good deal of hospital experience can earn up to $15 an hour. Pay scales vary in different regions of the country, however.

Interestingly, female technicians tend to make slightly more than male technicians. According to the *Pharmacy Week* salary survey, the median pay is $11.00 per hour for female technicians, and $10.35 for male technicians.

Pharmacy technicians who work in hospitals make more than technicians who work in community pharmacies: $11.70 an hour versus $9.25 an hour. This is probably because hospital technicians require more training and perform more difficult tasks, such as making IV solutions.

Pharmacy technicians who are certified also make about $2 more an hour than technicians who are not certified. Pharmacy technicians must pass a standardized test before they can become certified.

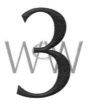

Preparing for a Career in Pharmacy

Pharmacists and pharmacy technicians should generally be people who like to help others. In addition, they should be able to work by themselves without a lot of supervision and should not mind doing repetitive tasks over and over again.

Pharmaceutical scientists, like any other scientists, should be very inquisitive and self-directed. They should like to investigate things and figure out why and how things happen. They should also be people who pay close attention to detail, and who do not mind spending long hours in a laboratory.

Pharmacists and pharmacy technicians also need to be very attentive to detail, because if patients are given the wrong medication by mistake, they could be seriously injured or even die. Unfortunately, mistakes do slip by occasionally, but pharmacists have to be very careful to avoid mistakes at all costs.

In addition to having the above qualities, pharmacists and pharmaceutical scientists must go through years and years of training. Pharmacy

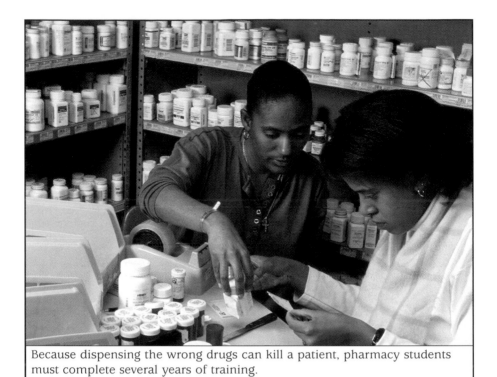
Because dispensing the wrong drugs can kill a patient, pharmacy students must complete several years of training.

technicians must also be trained for their work, but not for nearly as long as pharmacists or scientists. In this chapter, we'll look at what kind of education, training, and licensure you need to work as a pharmacist, a technician, or a pharmaceutical scientist.

Pharmacists

Pharmacists are licensed professionals. That means they must pass a national pharmacy licensing exam before they are granted a license to practice pharmacy. In addition, they must also pass a national pharmacy law exam and a state pharmacy law exam. But, before they are even allowed to sit for each of these exams, pharmacy students must first complete about six years of college.

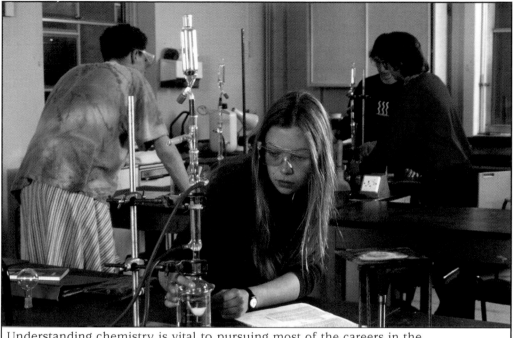

Understanding chemistry is vital to pursuing most of the careers in the pharmaceutical industry.

High School and College Preparation

For those of you who are now in high school and are interested in eventually going to pharmacy school, you should have good enough grades and a decent enough score on your SAT or ACT to get into college. It is not necessary to take advanced placement (AP) math or science classes in high school, although some students do so in order to get out of a few freshman-level classes in college.

Pre-pharmacy college classes include a large amount of math and science classes, so if you have the chance, you should take plenty of math and science classes in high school to prepare yourself. If you don't enjoy science at all, you may want to rethink your career choice at this point.

College Coursework

Although every university is different, most pharmacy schools require students to take about one or two years of pre-pharmacy courses before they are even allowed to apply to the pharmacy school itself. These pre-pharmacy courses usually include algebra, calculus, biology, physics, chemistry, organic chemistry, biochemistry, physiology, microbiology, and maybe human anatomy and cellular or molecular biology. In addition to these classes, students will also have to take the basic freshman and sophomore level classes that are required by their university, such as liberal arts and humanities classes.

Students generally apply to pharmacy school after the first year and a half of pre-pharmacy courses, but this depends on the school policy. Some students who change majors during college may find themselves applying to pharmacy school in the third year of college. Other pharmacy students even apply after they have already earned an undergraduate degree in another scientific discipline. However, the majority of students usually apply after the first year or two of college.

Applying to Pharmacy School and the PCAT Test

Since most pharmacy schools are within larger universities, students must first apply to the school before being admitted to the program. Although every pharmacy school is different, most schools accept students based on their college GPA, letters of reference, and sometimes a personal interview.

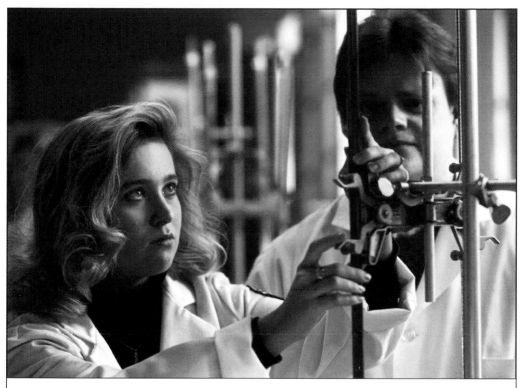
Pharmacy students must take and pass a variety of science courses to earn a degree.

Some but not all pharmacy schools require students to take the PCAT. PCAT stands for Pharmacy College Admissions Test. Since the PCAT tests students primarily on their knowledge of math and general sciences, students generally take the PCAT after taking their pre-pharmacy courses. A good place to find out more about the PCAT is on the Web site of the American Colleges of Clinical Pharmacy (ACCP) at http://www.aacp.org.

Pharmacy School

After being admitted to pharmacy school, usually in the third year of college, students finally get to take three or four years of actual pharmacy courses. These pharmacy courses include several semesters of pharmacy practice, pharmacology, pharmaceutics, organic medicinal chemistry, calculations, and therapeutics. In addition, most schools also offer courses in toxicology, biotechnology, therapeutics, geriatrics, and other specialized areas of interest.

In the first two or three years of academic courses, pharmacy students learn the basics, and are then assigned to clinical courses for their last year or two of pharmacy school. These courses are actual hands-on, in-hospital work, usually done in university hospitals or clinics.

Clinical courses are a most exciting time, because this is where all of your knowledge will finally come together. Pharmacy students get to work alongside physicians, pharmacists, nurses, medical students, and other allied health professions, in order to better learn how to take care of real patients.

On clinical rotations, pharmacy students go on rounds with the attending physicians and medical students. You'll usually be assigned patients of your own to monitor and ensure their drug therapies are appropriate. You'll also answer questions for doctors and medical students, and give presentations.

Internships

Many students must work in pharmacies as pharmacy interns during their years in pharmacy school. As pharmacy interns, students work alongside licensed pharmacists to gain valuable professional experience. Most states require that students spend 1,000 to 2,000 hours as pharmacy interns before they are granted their pharmacy licenses.

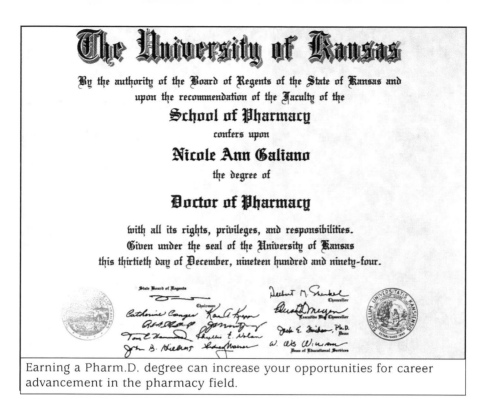

Earning a Pharm.D. degree can increase your opportunities for career advancement in the pharmacy field.

Graduation and Degrees Awarded

The two degrees currently awarded to pharmacists today are a five-year B.S. (bachelor of science) in pharmacy, and a six-year Pharm.D. (doctor of pharmacy) degree.

Presently, most of the eighty-one accredited U.S. schools of pharmacy award the Pharm.D. degree, and only a few still award only the B.S. degree. However, after 2005, all schools of pharmacy will be required to offer only the Pharm.D. degree.

Taking the "Boards" (the National Licensure Exam)

After graduation, pharmacy interns are finally allowed to "sit for the boards." The boards are two days of exams that consist of the national pharmacy licensing exam—called the NAPLEX—plus a federal pharmacy law exam—called the FDLE—plus a state pharmacy law exam.

Once you pass your boards, you will then be granted a pharmacy license from the state, or states, in which you want to practice. If you wish to practice in more than one state, you must take a separate pharmacy law test for each state you want to practice pharmacy in. This is due to the fact that pharmacy laws vary from state to state.

Keeping Your License Up to Date and in Good Standing

To keep your pharmacy license in good standing, you must pay a licensing fee to the state(s) in which you practice every one or two years. In addition to paying this fee, you must complete a certain amount of continuing education hours— usually about fifteen hours a year.

In addition to keeping your license current, you must also obey all the pharmacy laws and not participate in any illegal activities. Pharmacists who are caught participating in illegal drug activity or failing to practice pharmacy lawfully often end up losing their licenses or having them suspended.

Postgraduate Work

After graduation, some pharmacists decide to continue their education even further. They may decide to do an additional year of training at a hospital; this is called a residency. They may also go on to earn special certifications in an area of pharmacy that they are especially interested in, such as geriatrics or diabetes.

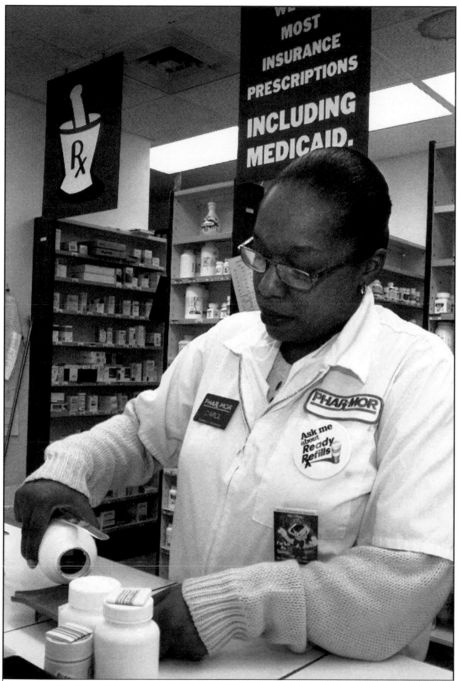

Pharmacy technicians often learn the field through on-the-job training as well as formal educational programs.

Pharmaceutical Scientists

Pharmaceutical scientists need more education than pharmacists. Most pharmaceutical scientists first earn a bachelor of science degree and then go on to earn a Ph.D. degree in their area of interest.

A pharmacologist may first earn a B.S. degree in pharmacy, and then go on to do his or her Ph.D. in pharmacology with a an emphasis on antibiotics. After earning a Ph.D., he or she may go on to do several years of postdoctoral training on antibiotic resistance to fluroquinolones—a specific class of antibiotics. So, as you can see, the work of a pharmaceutical scientist often gets very detailed and very specific.

Pharmacy Technicians

The most common way that people learn to become pharmacy technicians is through on-the-job-training. On-the-job training means that your employer will teach you everything you need to know as you learn how to do your job. There are also many formal educational programs that train pharmacy technicians throughout the country. These programs are usually offered through community colleges, technical institutes, or through the American Society of Health-System Pharmacists. (ASHP). The armed forces also offer formal training for pharmacy technicians.

According to the Pharmacy Technician Educators Council, students who attend pharmacy technician schools learn the names of medications, their actions, their common doses, and the reasons the medications are used. Pharmacy technician students also take classes in medical and pharmacy terminology, pharmacy communication skills, pharmaceutical calculations, pharmacy record keeping, and pharmacy law and ethics. Most training programs will award students either a certificate, a diploma, or an associate degree after they successfully complete the program.

Certification

In the 1990s, the Pharmacy Technician Certification Board began to offer a voluntary National Pharmacy Technician Certification Examination to pharmacy technicians. Not all technicians need to become certified, but certified technicians usually earn more than technicians who are not certified. Many employers will even pay the exam fee for their technicians to become certified.

To become certified, technicians must pass a national exam. In addition, technicians must complete a certain amount of continuing education every year in order to keep their certification. Most pharmacy technician training schools will help students to prepare for the certification test.

Registering with the State Board of Pharmacy

In many states, pharmacy technicians are required to register with the state, just as a pharmacist would, and pay an annual fee for a pharmacy technician license. Many states do a background check on pharmacy technicians, so if you have a history of criminal drug use or felony drug convictions, you most likely won't be granted a technician license.

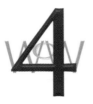

The Future of Pharmacy

There is an incredible shortage of pharmacists in the United States today. Because Americans are living longer, and older Americans tend to use more medications, the amount of prescriptions filled in pharmacies keeps increasing. Therefore, the need for pharmacists and pharmacy technicians will be around for quite a while.

But will the way pharmacy is practiced always be the same? Not necessarily. For years now, pharmacists have been moving away from the traditional dispensing role of pharmacists and focusing more on clinical duties. Some pharmacists today even prescribe medications in conjunction with doctors and hospitals. These days, pharmacy technicians are now doing most of the physical, dispensing work in pharmacies—a trend that will likely continue.

Advances in information technology are also making it a very interesting time for pharmacists. Pharmacists are now able to do more work much faster, and without always having to "be there" in person. For example, Internet pharmacies now allow patients to have their prescriptions filled over the

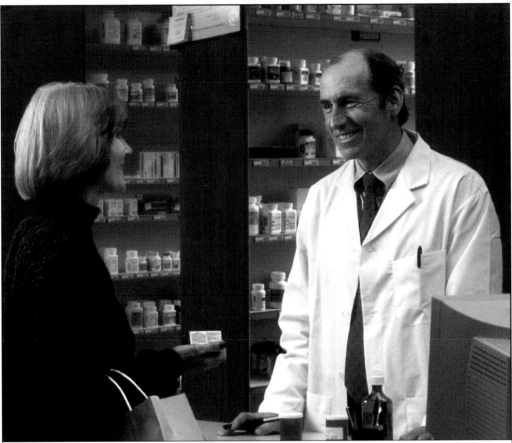

If you want to pursue a career as a pharmacist, it helps to have strong interpersonal skills because you will have to field many questions about the medications you dispense.

Internet, and e-mail their questions to the pharmacist. Computer software programs now allow pharmacists to check for potential drug interactions before a prescription is filled. Faxes and modern computer software in hospitals now allow nurses to obtain medications from pharmacy vending machines right there on the floor, without having to wait for them to come up from the pharmacy! And consultant and clinical pharmacists can now communicate with doctors and other health professionals via e-mail, instead of waiting all day for a phone call or a letter to be sent to them.

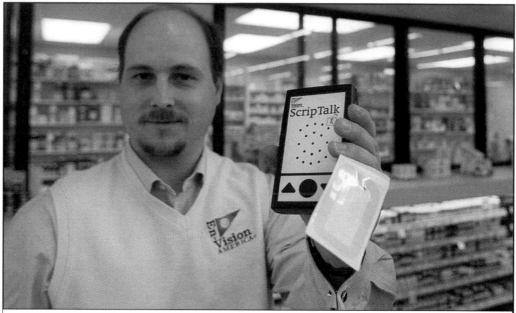

David Raistrick, vice president of En-Vision America, displays the ScripTalk Talking Prescription Reader, which enables sight-impaired people to hear spoken prescription instructions by pointing the device at a special label on a bottle of medication.

The information technology of the future might even be more amazing! Soon, doctors may have personal digital prescription machines that will connect directly to pharmacy computers. Or patients may someday get their medications from robotic pharmacy vending machines, instead of a pharmacist. Will all this new technology put pharmacists out of work? Probably not. Because even if the need for dispensing pharmacists is reduced, the need for clinical pharmacists could increase.

Advances in biotechnology will probably change pharmacy and the pharmaceutical sciences even more than advances in technology have. Now that the human genome has been completely mapped, biotechnology may completely change

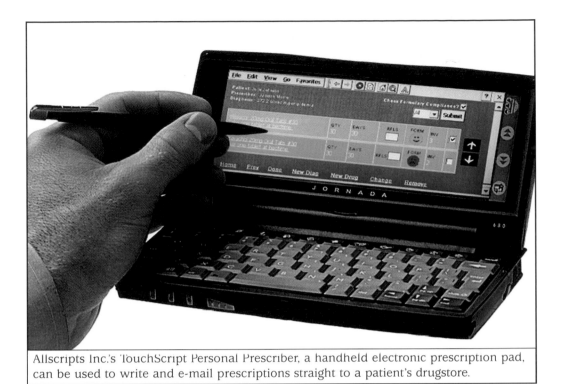

Allscripts Inc.'s TouchScript Personal Prescriber, a handheld electronic prescription pad, can be used to write and e-mail prescriptions straight to a patient's drugstore.

the way modern medicine is practiced. For example, instead of using medications to treat cancer or diabetes, pharmaceutical scientists may be able to create a way to change a person's DNA so that his or her body will not ever acquire cancer or diabetes in the first place! And instead of pharmacists and technicians dispensing pills or mixing IV medications, they may be mixing up gene therapy treatments for patients. Who knows—the possibilities are endless!

Where to Go from Here

If you love science and you are interested in helping people who are ill, pharmacy may be just the career you are looking for. The resources

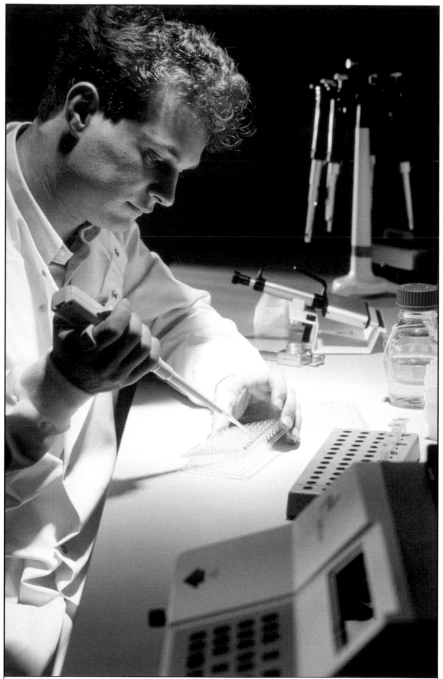

Recent advances in both technology and biotechnology will likely improve the way pharmaceuticals are researched and developed.

listed in the back of this book will provide you with additional information about careers in pharmacy and the training programs you will need to take in order to get started. There are many different careers in pharmacy, some of which require a good deal of college education and some that require little or no college education. One thing is for sure: There will always be a need for people to receive health care, so the future of pharmacy looks bright.

Glossary

antibiotic   Substance that destroys or slows the growth of bacteria or other microorganisms.

bacteria   A group of tiny organisms too small to be seen with the naked eye. Bacteria live all over our world: in soil, water, air, humans, animals, and plants. Most bacteria are not harmful, but some can cause disease by producing poisons in the body.

chart   A patient's hospital chart is a plastic folder that contains all the patient's important medical information. Different sections of a patient's chart include: medical history and physical exam; labs and X rays; doctor's progress notes; dietary and nutritional information; and pharmacy medication administration records.

dispense   To prepare and give medicine to patients.

drug allergy   Disorder in which the body becomes overly sensitive to a drug or medication. Symptoms can range from mild to severe.

drug interaction   A potentially harmful reaction that can occur in a person's body when two or more drugs or medications are taken at the same time.

drug therapy   Using drugs or medicines in order to treat or heal an illness in a patient.

ingest   When a food or other substance is chewed or swallowed and enters a patient's body.

IV   Stands for intravenous. When a drug is given as an IV, it is given intravenously, or into a person's vein. Once a medication is injected into a person's vein, it then goes directly into the patient's bloodstream. IV drugs are usually given when the patients are very sick, when they can't take pills, or when a drug is not available as a pill.

prescription   Written direction from a doctor to a pharmacist. A prescription tells a pharmacist what type and how much of a medicine to give to a patient.

radioactive   When a substance emits radiation, it is called a radioactive substance. Radiation is energy that is given off in the form of waves or particles, as a result of the molecule's nucleus disintegrating. Some of the common radioactive substances used in medicine and pharmacy are radioactive iodine, radioactive thallium, and radioactive cobalt.

residency   When a pharmacist or a medical doctor goes through a residency, that means they become a "resident" in a hospital for one or more years, and learn more about their profession. Residents are licensed professionals responsible for the care of their patients, but they work under the watchful eye of other, more experienced professionals who can help them learn.

toxicologist   Someone who studies toxicology. Toxicology is the study of poisonous materials and their effects upon living organisms.

For More Information

In the United States

American Association of Colleges of Pharmacy
1426 Prince Street
Alexandria, VA 22314
(703) 739-2330
Web site: http://www.aacp.org

American Institute of the History of Pharmacy
    at the University of Wisconsin School
    of Pharmacy
425 North Charter Street
Madison, WI 53706-1515
(608) 262-5378
Web site: http://www.pharmacy.wisc.edu/aihp
The institute publishes of a variety of interesting
books and booklets on the history of pharmacy
and medicine. For a list of books, click
on "publications."

American Pharmaceutical Association (APHA)
2215 Constitution Avenue NW
Washington, DC 20037-2985
(202) 628-4410
Web site: http://www.aphanet.org

American Society of Consultant Pharmacists
1321 Duke Street
Alexandria, VA 22314-3563
(703) 739-1300
Web site: http://www.ascp.com
The Web site contains valuable information about the job duties of consultant pharmacists.

American Society of Health-System Pharmacists
7272 Wisconsin Avenue
Bethesda, MD 20814
(301) 657-3000
Web site: http://www.ashp.org

Organizations for Pharmacy Technicians and Prospective Pharmacy Technicians

American Association of Pharmacy Technicians
P.O. Box 1447
Greensboro, NC 27402
(877) 368-4771
Web site: http://www.pharmacytechnician.com

National Certification for Pharmacy Technicians
    Technician Certification Board
2215 Constitution Avenue NW
Washington, DC 20037-2985
(202) 429-7576
Web site: http://www.ptcb.org
This is an excellent resource for pharmacy technicians interested in taking the certification exam. Contains valuable information about exam dates, costs, information, and practice tests.

Organizations for Pharmaceutical Scientists

American Association of Pharmaceutical
    Scientists (AAPS)
2107 Wilson Boulevard, Suite 700
Arlington, VA 22201-3046
(703) 243-2800
Web site: http://www.aapspharmaceutica.com

In Canada

For a complete list of Canadian and international schools of pharmacy, you can access the official world list of pharmacy schools Web page at
http://www.cf.ac.uk/phrmy/WWW-WSP/
    SoPListHomePage.html

Web Sites

Association of Natural Medicine Pharmacists
http://www.anmp.org
This is an interesting Web site for pharmacists who are interested in natural medicine, such as herbs and plants.

History of Pharmacy
http://www.pharmacy.wsu.edu/history
Provides an interesting look at the history of pharmacy.

PharmacyOneSource
http://www.pharmacyonesource.com
Provides information about jobs, student resources, colleges, and technician training programs.

Pharmacy Week
http://www.pharmacyweek.com
Gives you an insight into the types of jobs that are available. Contains valuable information about pharmacy salaries.

For Further Reading

Gable, Fred B. *Opportunities in Pharmacy Careers.* Lincolnwood, IL: VGM Career Horizons, 1998.

James, Robert. *Pharmacists: People Who Care for Our Health.* Vero Beach, FL: Rourke Book Company, 1995.

Stonier, Peter D., ed. *Discovering New Medicines: Careers in Pharmaceutical Research and Development.* New York: John Wiley and Sons, 1995.

Index

About the Author

Nicole (Niki) Galiano, Pharm.D., has been a registered pharmacist since graduating from the University of Kansas in 1993. After graduating with her B.S. in pharmacy, she went on to earn her Pharm.D. degree in 1994, also from the University of Kansas. Most of her professional experience has been in the area of hospital pharmacy, but she has also worked as a long-term care pharmacist, a retail/community pharmacist, a home infusion pharmacist, a clinical drug trial pharmacist, and as an educational program manager for a national pharmacy association. Currently, Niki is working as a traveling/relief pharmacist in the Kansas City area.

If you have any questions for Niki about careers in pharmacy, you can reach her at nikiano@earthlink.net.

Photo Credits

Cover, pp. 7, 9, 18, 23, 31, 39, 41, 49 © Corbis; pp. 2, 12, 38, 52 © Index Stock; pp. 28, 33, 45, 50, 51 © AP/Wide World Photos; p. 43 by Dean Galiano.

Design

Nelson Sá